K.A. DIESEL

# Chair Yoga for Seniors

*Reduce Stress, Lose Weight and Increase Flexibility*

This book was professionally typeset on Reedsy.
Find out more at reedsy.com

# Contents

# 1

# Introduction

First, this book is meant to be introductory into the world of chair yoga for seniors. The hope is that this book will provide you the basics to work on in an effort to excel to higher levels. I want to congratulate you for picking up this book and taking this step towards reclaiming your health and well-being. In this book, I'll guide you through the practice of chair yoga, offering tailored advice to address unique mobility needs and challenges. Regardless of your current condition or experience with yoga, this book aims to make yoga accessible to all. So, let's embark on this journey together and reclaim our vitality. In a world where age often dictates our limitations, the notion of vitality can seem like a distant dream. Yet, within the realm of chair yoga lies a pathway to rejuvenation and well-being, regardless of age or physical condition.

Consider this: A recent survey found that nearly 80% of seniors struggle with mobility issues, leading to a decline in quality of life. However, amidst these challenges, there exists a beacon of hope - chair yoga.

According to data from the National Institutes of Health, regular practice of chair yoga has been linked to significant improvements in balance, flexibility, and overall mental well-being among seniors. But beyond the numbers, lies a deeper truth: the transformative power of chair yoga extends far beyond physical exercise.

Imagine waking up each day feeling stronger, more flexible, and mentally resilient. That's the promise of chair yoga. By embarking on this journey, you're not just reclaiming your mobility; you're reclaiming your life.

# 2

# Understanding Chair Yoga

The Essence of Chair Yoga: A Path to Enhanced Well-Being

Chair yoga, often overlooked in the realm of traditional yoga practices, offers a gentle yet profound approach to enhancing overall well-being. Unlike its more vigorous counterparts, chair yoga is practiced sitting on a chair or using a chair for support, making it accessible to individuals of all ages and physical abilities. At its core, chair yoga emphasizes the integration of breath, movement, and mindfulness, fostering a deeper connection between body and mind. Through a series of gentle stretches, twists, and mindful breathing exercises, chair yoga offers a pathway to increased flexibility, improved posture, and enhanced mental clarity.

**Why Chair Yoga is Perfect for Seniors**

For seniors, chair yoga serves as a beacon of hope amidst the challenges of aging. As we age, our bodies undergo various changes, leading to reduced mobility, flexibility, and strength. However, chair yoga offers a tailored approach to fitness, addressing common physical limitations while providing a gentle yet effective means of maintaining overall health. Through regular practice, seniors can experience improvements in balance, flexibility, and mental well-being, ultimately leading to a higher quality of life.

**Overcoming Mobility Barriers with Chair Yoga**

One of the greatest barriers to physical activity among seniors is limited mobility that can impede their ability to engage in physical activity and maintain independence. Common mobility challenges include stiffness in joints, reduced range of motion, muscle weakness, and balance issues. However, chair yoga offers a gentle and accessible way to overcome these barriers and improve mobility. Through modified poses and gentle movements, chair yoga enables individuals with mobility issues to reap the benefits of yoga without the fear of injury or strain. By gradually building strength and flexibility, seniors can overcome mobility barriers and regain confidence in their bodies.

Research studies have consistently shown positive results from a daily regimen of chair yoga for seniors with mobility issues. A study published in the *Journal of Aging and Physical Activity* found that participants who engaged in regular chair yoga sessions experienced significant improvements in flexibility, balance, and functional mobility after just eight weeks. Another study published in the *International Journal of Yoga Therapy* reported similar findings, with participants showing increased mobility and reduced pain levels following a consistent chair yoga practice.

Specific poses and movements in chair yoga target key areas of mobility, such as the spine, hips, shoulders, and ankles. Gentle stretches and range-of-motion exercises help to lubricate the joints, release tension in muscles, and improve flexibility. Additionally, balancing poses and weight-bearing exercises strengthen the muscles that support mobility and stability.

By incorporating chair yoga into their daily routine, seniors can gradually overcome mobility barriers and experience greater freedom of movement and independence. With regular practice and dedication, chair yoga has the potential to enhance overall mobility, reduce the risk of falls, and improve quality of life for seniors.

## Setting Realistic Goals with Chair Yoga

In the journey towards wellness, setting realistic goals is paramount. Chair yoga provides a platform for individuals to set personalized goals based on their unique needs and abilities. Whether it's improving flexibility, reducing stress, or enhancing overall well-being, chair yoga offers a flexible and adaptable approach to goal setting.

While every individual's body responds differently to regular practice, it's essential to understand that chair yoga is a gradual process that yields long-term benefits. On average, seniors can expect to start noticing positive results from a daily practice routine of chair yoga within 4 to 8 weeks.

Initially, you may experience subtle changes in your flexibility, mobility, and overall sense of well-being. These changes may manifest as increased ease in everyday movements, reduced stiffness in joints, and a greater sense of relaxation and mental clarity.

As you continue with your daily chair yoga practice, these improvements are likely to become more pronounced. You may notice significant gains in flexibility, strength, and balance, as well as a reduction in stress levels and improved quality of sleep.

It's important to approach your chair yoga practice with patience, consistency, and an open mind. Progress may not always be linear, and there may be days when you feel less flexible or energetic than others. However, by staying committed to your practice and trusting in the process, you will gradually see positive changes unfold over time.

Remember, the journey of chair yoga is not just about achieving specific physical goals but also about cultivating a deeper connection with yourself and your body. Celebrate each milestone along the way and be kind to yourself as you navigate the ups and downs of your practice. With dedication and perseverance, chair yoga has the potential to transform not only your body but also your mind and spirit.

**Safety First: Pre-Yoga Health Checks**

Before embarking on any new exercise regimen, it's essential to prioritize safety. Chair yoga is no exception. Before beginning a chair yoga practice, seniors should consult with their healthcare provider to ensure that it is safe for them to do so. Additionally, individuals should be mindful of their own physical limitations and listen to their bodies during practice. By practicing proper warm-up techniques and paying attention to any signs of discomfort, seniors can minimize the risk of injury and maximize the benefits of chair yoga. I will be offering warm-up suggestions later on.

3

# Preparing for Chair Yoga

Before delving into the transformative practice of chair yoga, it's essential to lay the groundwork for a safe and enjoyable experience. In this chapter, we'll explore the key elements of preparation, including selecting the right equipment, understanding the importance of nutrition and hydration, and tuning into your body's signals.

**Choosing the Right Chair: Safety and Comfort**

Selecting the appropriate chair for chair yoga is crucial to ensure safety, stability, and comfort during practice. Here are examples of what to look for in a good chair versus what to avoid:

Good Chair:

- Flat, Firm Seat: Look for a chair with a flat, firm seat that provides a stable foundation for your practice.
- Backrest for Support: A chair with a backrest offers additional support, especially during seated poses and transitions.
- Stable Legs: Ensure the chair has sturdy legs that provide stability

and prevent tipping during movement.

- Armless Design: Chairs without arms allow for greater freedom of movement and accommodate a wider range of poses.

Bad Chair:

- Unstable Legs: Avoid chairs with wobbly or uneven legs, as they can compromise safety and stability during practice.
- Wheels: Chairs with wheels are not suitable for chair yoga practice, as they can move unexpectedly and cause accidents.
- Narrow Seat: Chairs with narrow or overly cushioned seats may not provide adequate support or stability during poses.
- Armrests: Chairs with armrests can restrict movement and hinder proper alignment during practice.

When choosing a chair for chair yoga practice, prioritize safety, stability, and comfort to ensure an enjoyable and beneficial experience. Avoid chairs with features that may impede movement or compromise safety, and opt for a sturdy, supportive chair that allows for freedom of movement and proper alignment.

**Yoga Equipment: Enhancements or Necessities?**

When it comes to chair yoga, the need for specialized equipment is minimal. While certain yoga props can enhance your practice, they are not always necessary, especially for beginners or those practicing at home. Here are some examples of household objects that can serve as alternatives to traditional yoga equipment:

Yoga Blocks:

- Home Alternative: Thick Books or Sturdy Pillows
- Thick books, such as dictionaries or encyclopedias, can be stacked to create a makeshift yoga block.
- Sturdy pillows or cushions can also be used to support and modify poses, providing comfort and stability.

Yoga Straps:

- Home Alternative: Towels or Belts
- A towel or belt can be used to facilitate stretches and provide support during poses that require reaching or stretching beyond your natural range of motion.
- Simply loop the towel or belt around your foot or hold onto it with your hands to deepen the stretch.

Yoga Blankets:

- Home Alternative: Thick Blankets or Towels
- Thick blankets or towels can be folded and used as padding or support under knees, hips, or other sensitive areas during seated or reclined poses.
- They can also provide warmth and comfort during relaxation and meditation practices.

Yoga Bolsters:

- Home Alternative: Rolled-Up Blankets or Pillows
- Rolled-up blankets or pillows can serve as makeshift bolsters to support the spine, neck, or knees during restorative poses.
- Adjust the thickness and firmness of the roll to suit your comfort and support needs.

Yoga Mat:

- Home Alternative: Non-Slip Rug or Carpet
- A non-slip rug or carpet can provide traction and stability during chair yoga practice, preventing the chair from sliding or shifting on smooth surfaces.
- Choose a textured or grippy surface that offers traction and support for your practice.

By utilizing household objects as alternatives to traditional yoga equipment, you can adapt your practice to suit your needs and preferences without investing in expensive props. Get creative and explore different options to find what works best for you, making your chair yoga practice accessible, enjoyable, and fulfilling.

**What to Wear: Comfort Meets Functionality**

When it comes to attire for chair yoga, prioritize comfort and functionality. Choose loose-fitting clothing that allows for ease of movement and breathability. Avoid garments with restrictive seams or fabrics that may impede mobility. Additionally, consider the temperature of your practice space and dress accordingly to ensure optimal comfort throughout your session.

**Warm-Up: Preparing Your Body for Yoga**

Before diving into your chair yoga practice, take a few moments to warm up your body. Simple stretching exercises and gentle movements can help prepare your muscles and joints for the practice ahead. Focus on areas of tension or stiffness, gradually easing into each movement with mindful awareness of your body's capabilities.

Seniors may have various physical limitations that require special attention and modifications during their practice. Here are some common senior physical limitations and suggested warm-ups tailored to address these limitations:

- **Limited Range of Motion in the Shoulders and Upper Body:** Seniors with limited shoulder mobility may benefit from gentle shoulder warm-up exercises to increase flexibility and range of motion. Example warm-up exercises include shoulder rolls, arm circles, and shoulder stretches using a towel or strap for assistance.

- **Stiffness and Tightness in the Lower Back**: Seniors experiencing stiffness or tightness in the lower back can benefit from warm-up exercises that gently mobilize the spine and release tension in the muscles surrounding the lumbar region. Examples include seated spinal twists, gentle seated forward folds, and pelvic tilts.

- **Decreased Flexibility in the Hips and Hamstrings**: Seniors with limited flexibility in the hips and hamstrings may find it beneficial to incorporate warm-up exercises that target these areas. Examples include seated hip circles, knee-to-chest stretches, and seated hamstring stretches with the legs extended or bent.

- **Reduced Balance and Stability**: Seniors who struggle with balance and stability can benefit from warm-up exercises that focus on improving proprioception and strengthening the muscles involved in balance. Examples include seated leg lifts, ankle circles, and toe taps to the floor while seated.

· **Arthritis or Joint Pain**: Seniors with arthritis or joint pain may require gentle warm-up exercises that help to lubricate the joints and reduce discomfort. Examples include gentle wrist and ankle circles, wrist flexion and extension exercises, and gentle range-of-motion movements for the knees and hips.

**Importance of Hydration and Nutrition**

Hydration and nutrition are essential pillars of overall health and well-being, providing the foundation for optimal energy levels, physical performance, and recovery. Adequate hydration and nourishing foods play a crucial role in supporting chair yoga practice and promoting vitality. Here's a breakdown of recommended daily water intake and examples of nourishing meals and snacks:

*Recommended Daily Water Intake:*
The recommended daily water intake for adults varies depending on factors such as age, gender, weight, and activity level. As a general guideline, it's recommended that adults aim to consume approximately 64 ounces (or 8 cups) of water per day. However, individual hydration needs may vary, so it's essential to listen to your body and adjust your water intake accordingly, especially if you're engaging in physical activity like chair yoga.

*Nourishing Food Examples for Sustained Energy and Muscle Recovery*

Breakfast:

- Example: Greek Yogurt Parfait
- Ingredients: Greek yogurt, mixed berries, granola, honey
- Benefits:  Greek yogurt provides protein for muscle repair and recovery, while mixed berries offer antioxidants and fiber. Granola adds crunch and complex carbohydrates for sustained energy, and a drizzle of honey adds natural sweetness.

Lunch:

- Example: Quinoa Salad with Chickpeas and Veggies
- Ingredients: Cooked quinoa, chickpeas, mixed vegetables (such as bell peppers, cucumber, cherry tomatoes), fresh herbs, olive oil, lemon juice, salt, pepper
- Benefits: Quinoa is a complete protein source, providing essential amino acids for muscle repair and growth.  Chickpeas offer additional protein and fiber, while mixed vegetables provide vitamins, minerals, and antioxidants. Olive oil adds healthy fats, and lemon juice adds flavor and vitamin C.

Snack:

- Example: Apple Slices with Almond Butter
- Ingredients: Apple slices, almond butter
- Benefits: Apples are a good source of fiber and natural sugars for a quick energy boost. Almond butter provides healthy fats, protein, and magnesium, which can support muscle function and recovery.

Dinner:

- Example: Baked Salmon with Roasted Vegetables
- Ingredients: Salmon fillet, mixed vegetables (such as broccoli, carrots, Brussels sprouts), olive oil, garlic, lemon, salt, pepper
- Benefits: Salmon is rich in omega-3 fatty acids, which have anti-inflammatory properties and support heart health. Mixed vegetables provide fiber, vitamins, and minerals, while olive oil and garlic add flavor and additional health benefits.

By incorporating hydrating fluids and nourishing foods into your daily routine, you can fuel your body for optimal performance and recovery, both on and off the yoga mat. Remember to prioritize hydration and nutrition as essential components of your chair yoga practice, supporting your overall health and well-being for years to come.

**Understanding Your Body's Signals**

As you engage in chair yoga, it's essential to tune into your body's signals and respond accordingly. Pay attention to any sensations of discomfort or strain, and modify or release poses as needed to ensure safety and comfort. Remember, yoga is a practice of self-awareness and self-care, so listen to your body's wisdom and honor its needs throughout your practice.

4

# Basic Poses and Modifications

I n the realm of chair yoga, simplicity meets potency. As we delve into this chapter, we'll explore a range of foundational poses designed to nurture flexibility, strength, and relaxation. From gentle upper body stretches to core-strengthening exercises, each pose offers a unique opportunity to connect with your body and breath.

**Introduction to Chair Yoga Poses**

Chair yoga poses are accessible to individuals of all ages and abilities, offering a gentle yet effective means of improving overall well-being. By practicing yoga while seated or using a chair for support, you can reap the benefits of this ancient practice without the need for complicated transitions or advanced postures. Each movement, and each pose should have a corresponding breath in the nose and out the mouth. Each breath represents a movement. Let's begin our journey into the world of chair yoga poses.

**Upper Body Stretches for Flexibility and Strength**

The upper body carries the weight of daily stress and tension, making it essential to incorporate stretches that promote flexibility and strength. From shoulder rolls to chest openers, these gentle stretches target key areas of tension, allowing you to release tightness and restore mobility.

Incorporating upper body stretches into your chair yoga practice can help improve flexibility, mobility, and strength in the arms, shoulders, chest, and upper back. Here are some effective poses and stretches to target the upper body:

**Seated Cat-Cow Stretch:**

- Begin seated on the edge of your chair with your feet flat on the floor and hands resting on your thighs.
- Inhale as you arch your spine, lifting your chest and drawing your shoulder blades together (Cow Pose).
- Exhale as you round your spine, tucking your chin to your chest and drawing your belly button towards your spine (Cat Pose).
- Repeat this fluid movement, syncing your breath with the movement of your spine, for several rounds to warm up the upper back and shoulders.

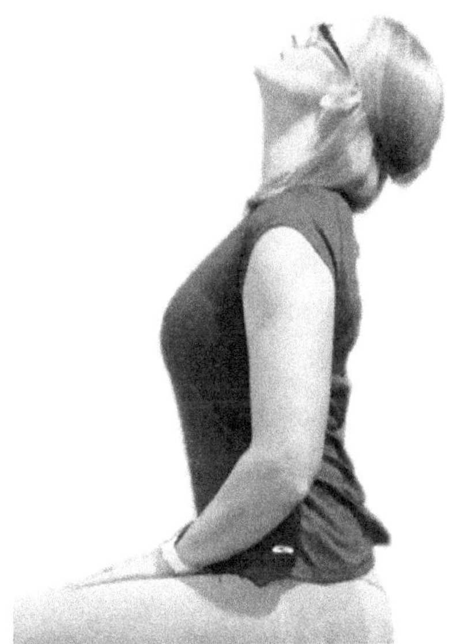 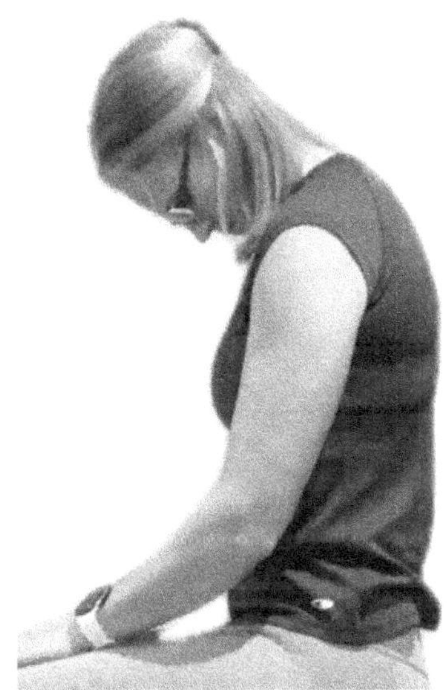

Modification suggestions:

- For individuals with arthritis in the wrists or hands, perform the movement with fingers lightly touching the chair seat instead of placing palms flat.
- Limit the range of motion if there's discomfort, moving only as far as feels comfortable and avoiding any sharp pain.

**Seated Shoulder Stretch:**

- Sit tall in your chair with your feet flat on the floor.
- Inhale and reach your right arm across your body, placing your left hand on your right elbow.
- Exhale and gently pull your right arm towards your chest until you feel a stretch in your right shoulder and upper back.
- Hold the stretch for 20-30 seconds, then switch sides and repeat on the left side.

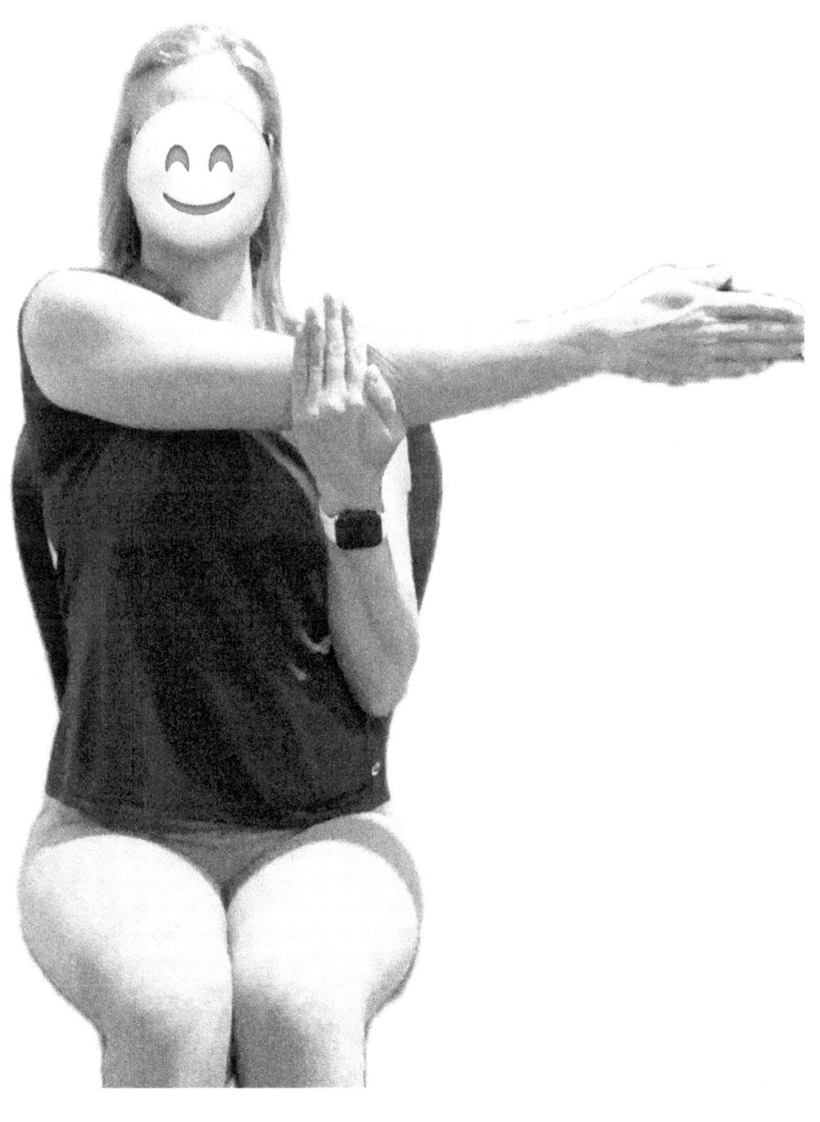

Seated Shoulder Stretch – Modifications:

- Use a towel or strap to assist in reaching the arm across the body if mobility is limited.
- Adjust the intensity of the stretch by gently pressing on the elbow, avoiding excessive force.

**Seated Eagle Arms:**

- Sit tall in your chair and extend your arms straight out in front of you at shoulder height.
- Inhale and cross your right arm over your left, bringing your palms to touch if possible.
- Exhale and lift your elbows slightly and press your palms away from your face, feeling a stretch across the upper back and shoulders.
- Hold the pose for 20-30 seconds, then release and switch sides, crossing your left arm over your right.

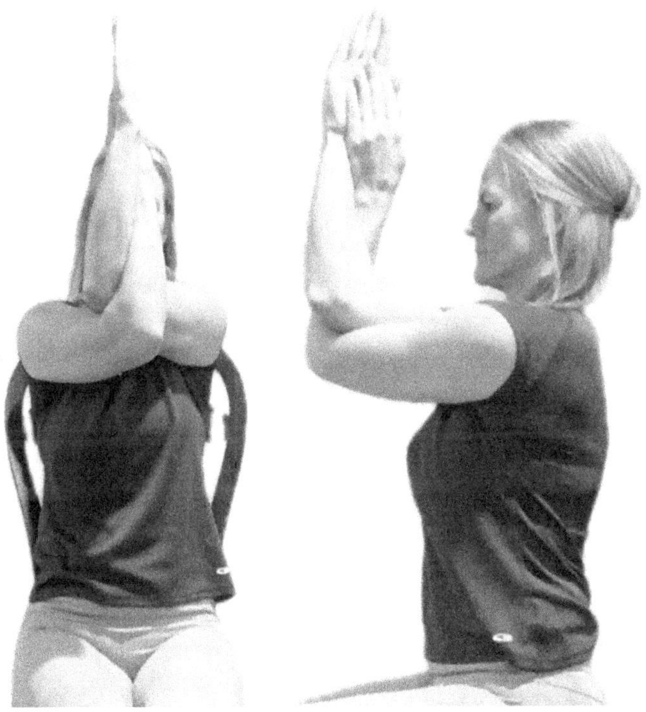

Seated Eagle Arms - Modifications:

- If crossing the arms is challenging, simply bring the arms parallel to each other in front of the body and hold in a comfortable position.
- Focus on drawing the shoulder blades together and maintaining good posture to engage the upper back muscles.

**Seated Chest Opener:**

- Sit tall in your chair with your feet flat on the floor and interlace your fingers behind your lower back.

- Inhale and press your palms together and straighten your arms, lifting your hands away from your body.
- Exhale and draw your shoulder blades together and lift your chest towards the ceiling, feeling a stretch across the front of your chest and shoulders.
- Hold the pose for 20-30 seconds, breathing deeply into the stretch.

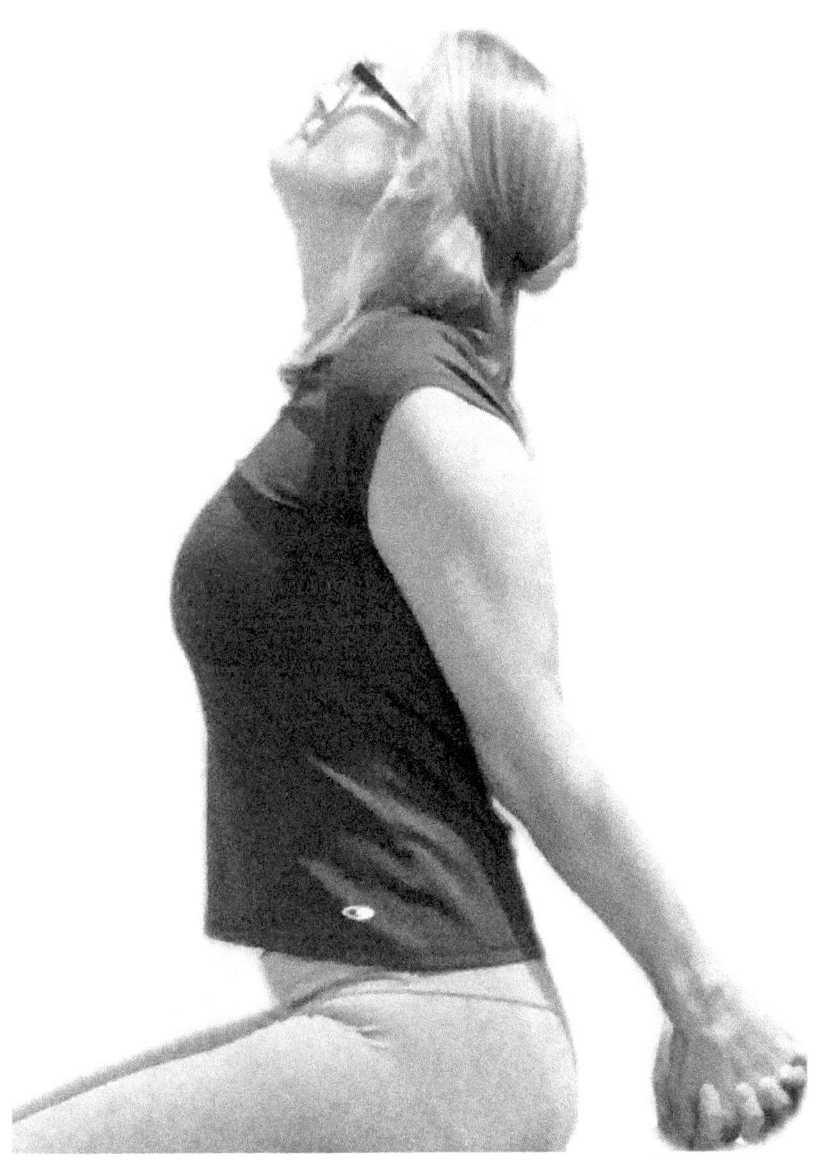

Seated Chest Opener – Modifications:

- Individuals with shoulder or upper back issues can modify it by bringing the hands to the sides of the backrest of the chair or clasping hands behind the back at a comfortable level.
- Focus on opening the chest gently, avoiding any strain in the shoulders or upper back.

**Seated Tricep Stretch:**

- Sit tall in your chair, inhale and reach your right arm overhead, bending your elbow and placing your palm on the center of your upper back.
- Use your left hand to gently press on your right elbow, exhale while deepening the stretch in your right tricep.
- Hold the stretch for 20-30 seconds, then switch sides and repeat on the left side.

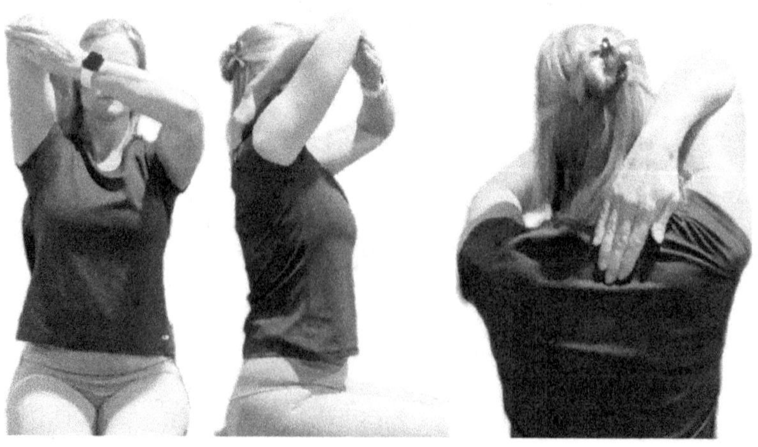

Seated Tricep Stretch – Modifications:

- If reaching the arm overhead is difficult, use the opposite hand to gently guide the elbow towards the center of the back.
- Adjust the stretch by varying the pressure applied to the elbow, ensuring it's comfortable and pain-free.

Incorporate these upper body stretches into your chair yoga practice to improve flexibility, mobility, and strength in your arms, shoulders, and upper back. Remember to breathe deeply and mindfully as you move through each stretch, listening to your body and honoring its needs and limitations.

By repeating these stretches, and poses, on a daily basis you will soon begin to see results in your mobility.

## Lower Body Work: Safe Leg and Foot Exercises

Maintaining mobility in the lower body is vital for overall functionality and independence. With a focus on safe leg and foot exercises, you can improve circulation, balance, and range of motion. From ankle circles to seated leg lifts, these exercises offer a gentle yet effective way to strengthen and tone the lower body.

Incorporating safe leg and foot exercises into your chair yoga practice can help improve lower body strength, flexibility, and mobility while reducing the risk of injury. Here are some effective poses and stretches to target the lower body:

**Seated Knee Lifts:**

- Sit tall in your chair with your feet flat on the floor.

- Hold onto the sides of your chair for support.
- Inhale and lift your right foot off the floor, bringing your knee towards your chest.
- Hold for a few seconds, then exhale and lower your foot back down.
- Repeat on the left side.
- Aim for 10-15 repetitions on each side, gradually increasing as you build strength.

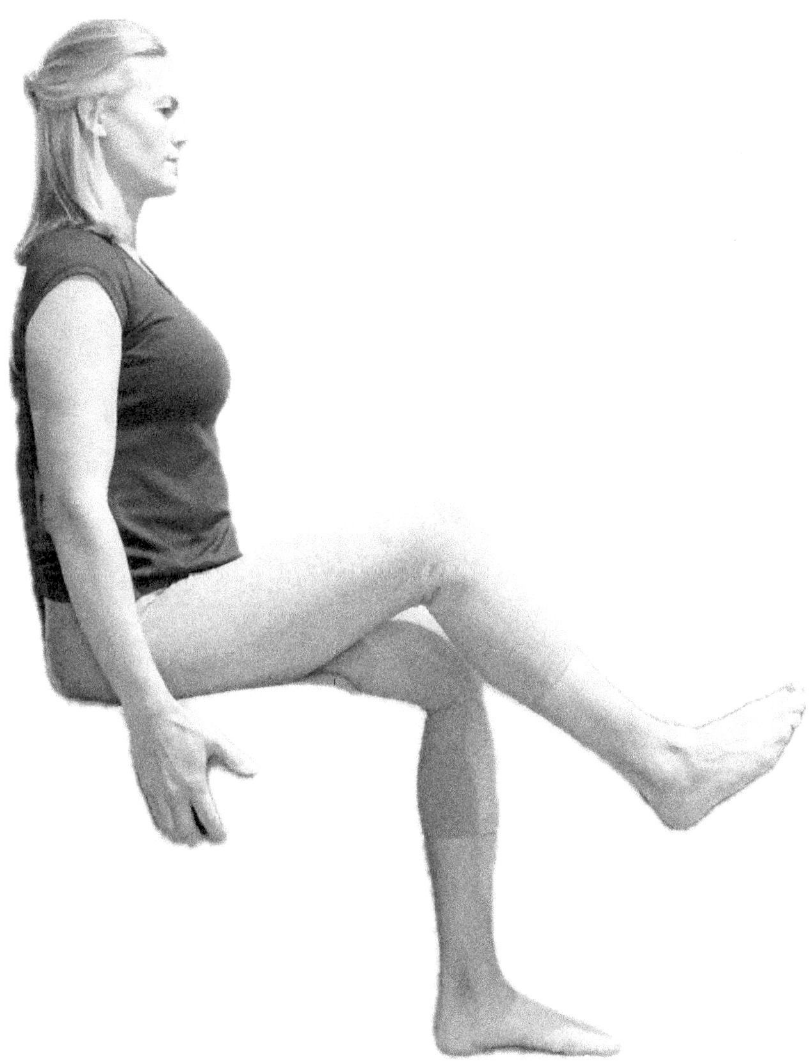

## Seated Leg Extensions:

- Sit tall in your chair with your feet flat on the floor.
- Inhale and extend your right leg straight out in front of you, keeping

your foot flexed.

- Exhale and hold for a few seconds, then bend your knee to bring your foot back to the floor.
- Repeat on the left side.
- Aim for 10-15 repetitions on each side, focusing on controlled movement and maintaining good posture.

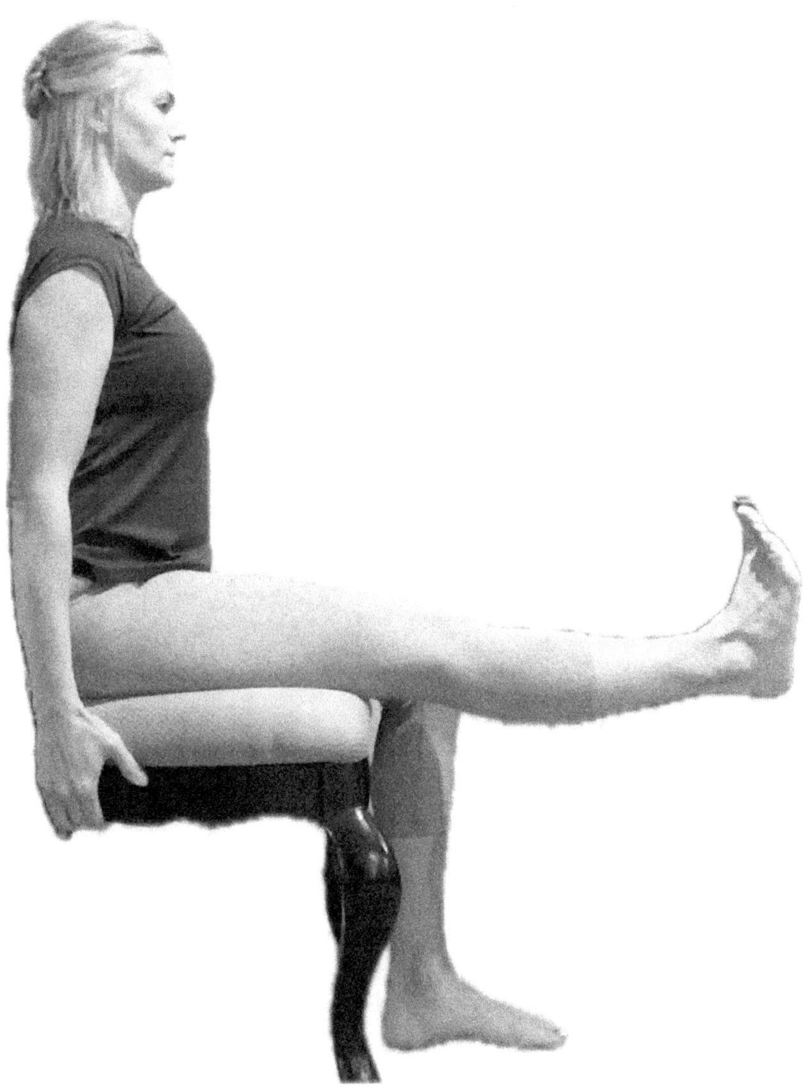

**Seated Figure-Four Stretch (slightly advanced):**

- Sit tall in your chair with your feet flat on the floor.
- Inhale and cross your right ankle over your left knee, creating a figure-four shape with your legs.
- Flex your right foot to protect your knee joint.
- Exhale and gently press down on your right knee to deepen the stretch in your right hip and outer thigh.
- Hold the stretch for 20-30 seconds, then switch sides and repeat on the left side.

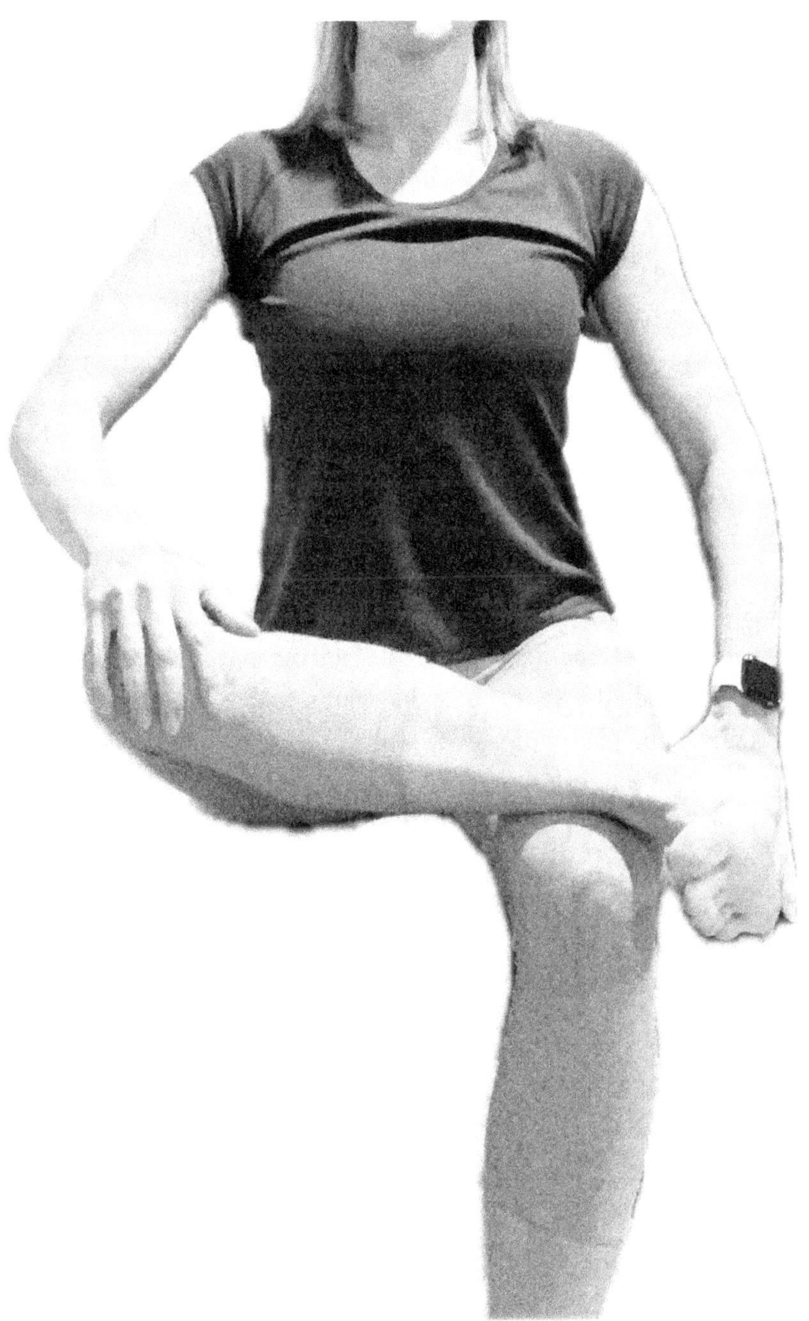

## Seated Figure-Four Stretch Modification:

- For individuals with knee or hip issues, limit the range of motion by hugging the knee towards the chest only as far as feels comfortable.
- As your flexibility and mobility increase over time, eventually you may find that you are able to place your right ankle over your left knee, and vice versa.
- Use the hands to support the leg if needed, avoiding any strain in the lower back or hips.

## Seated Calf Stretch:

- Sit tall in your chair with your feet flat on the floor.
- Inhale and extend your right leg straight out in front of you, keeping your heel on the floor and flexing your toes towards your body.
- Exhale and gently press down on your right knee to deepen the stretch in your calf muscle.
- Hold the stretch for 20-30 seconds, then switch sides and repeat on the left side.

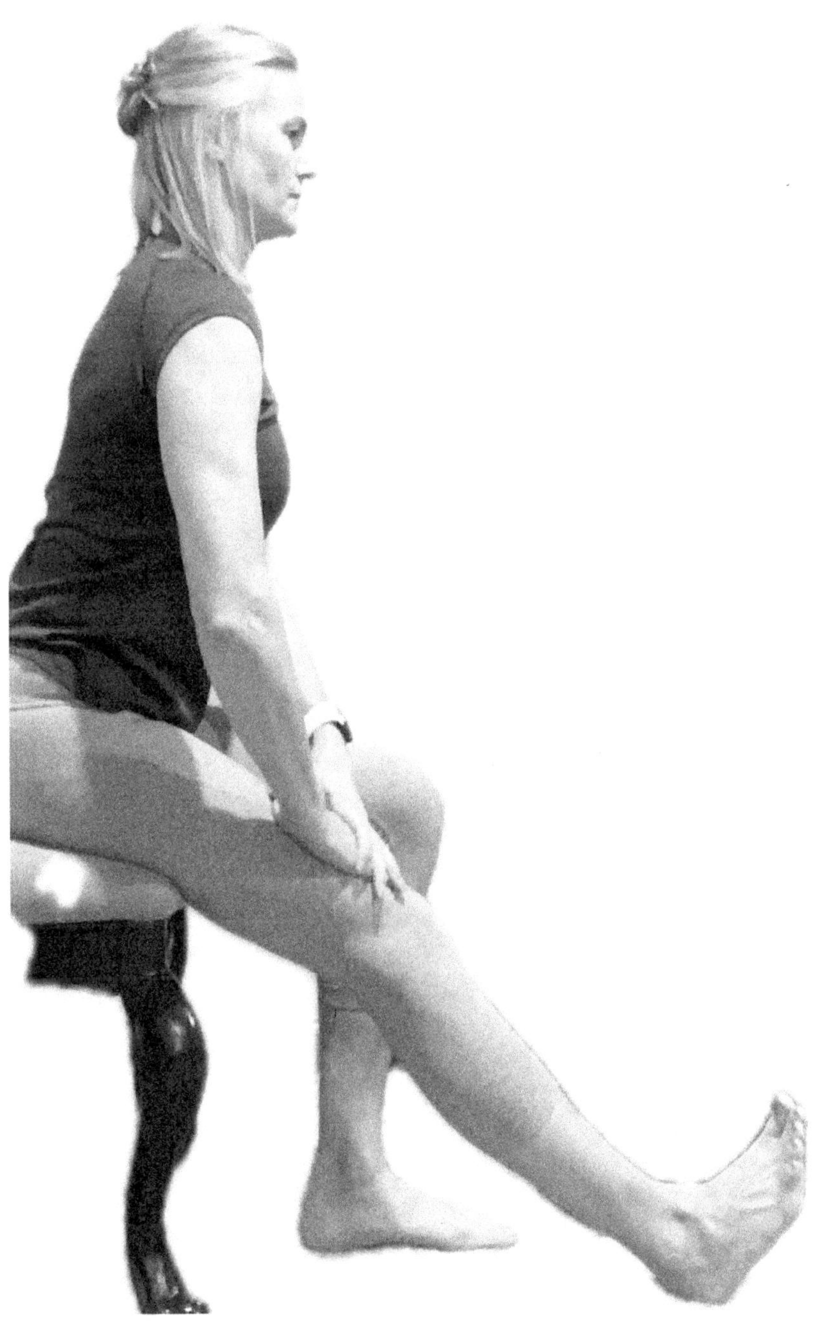

**Seated Ankle Circles:**

- Sit tall in your chair with your feet flat on the floor.
- Inhale and lift your right foot off the floor, exhale and circle your ankle clockwise for several rotations.
- Then, circle your ankle counterclockwise for several rotations.
- Repeat on the left side.
- Aim for 10-15 rotations in each direction on each side, focusing on smooth and controlled movement.

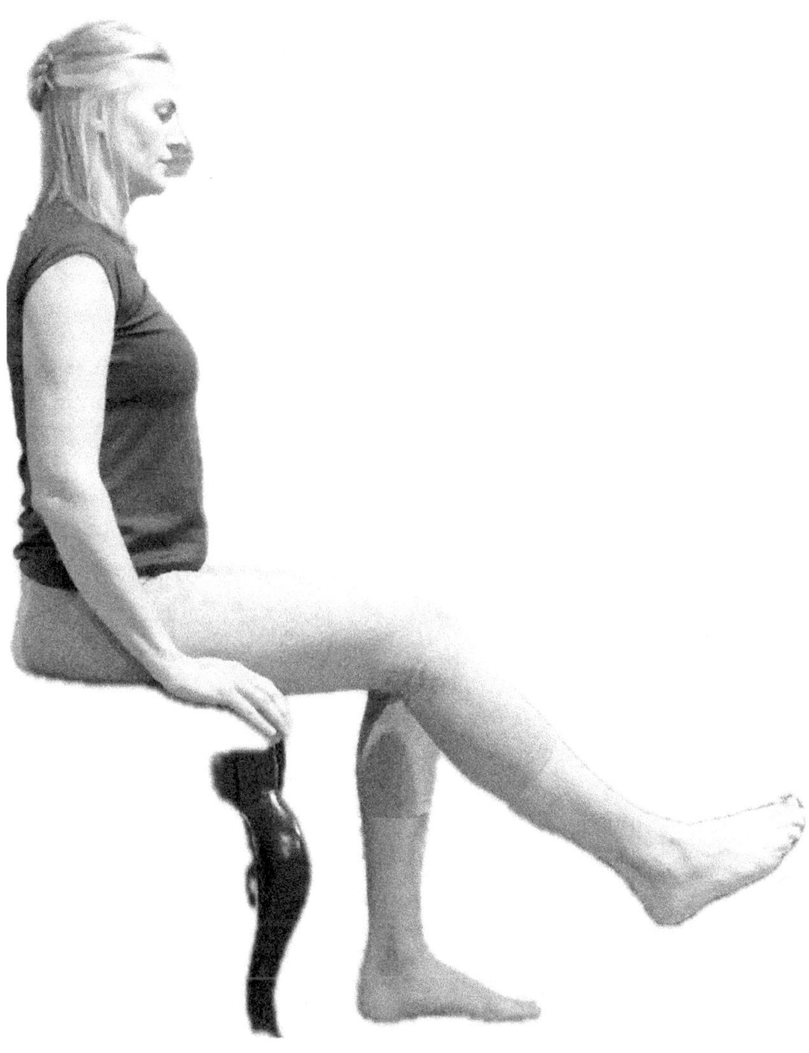

Incorporate these safe leg and foot exercises into your chair yoga practice to improve lower body strength, flexibility, and mobility. Remember to move mindfully and listen to your body, modifying or skipping any movements that cause pain or discomfort. With consistent practice, you can gradually build strength and flexibility in your lower body, enhancing your overall well-being and mobility.

## Core Strengthening Without the Strain

A strong core is the foundation of stability and balance, essential components of overall well-being. Through a series of core-strengthening exercises, and breath focus, you can build strength and stability without the strain of traditional abdominal workouts. From seated twists to pelvic tilts, these exercises engage the core muscles while promoting proper alignment and posture.

Strengthening the core muscles is essential for stability, balance, and posture, but it's important to do so without placing undue strain on the body, especially for seniors. Here are some gentle chair yoga poses and stretches that target the core muscles effectively without causing strain:

## Seated Spinal Twist:

- Sit tall in your chair with your feet flat on the floor.
- Place your right hand on the back of the chair and your left hand on your right thigh.
- Inhale to lengthen your spine, then exhale as you twist your torso to the right, looking over your right shoulder.
- Hold the twist for a few breaths, feeling the engagement in your core muscles.
- Inhale to return to center, then repeat on the other side.
- Aim for 3-5 repetitions on each side, moving slowly and with control.

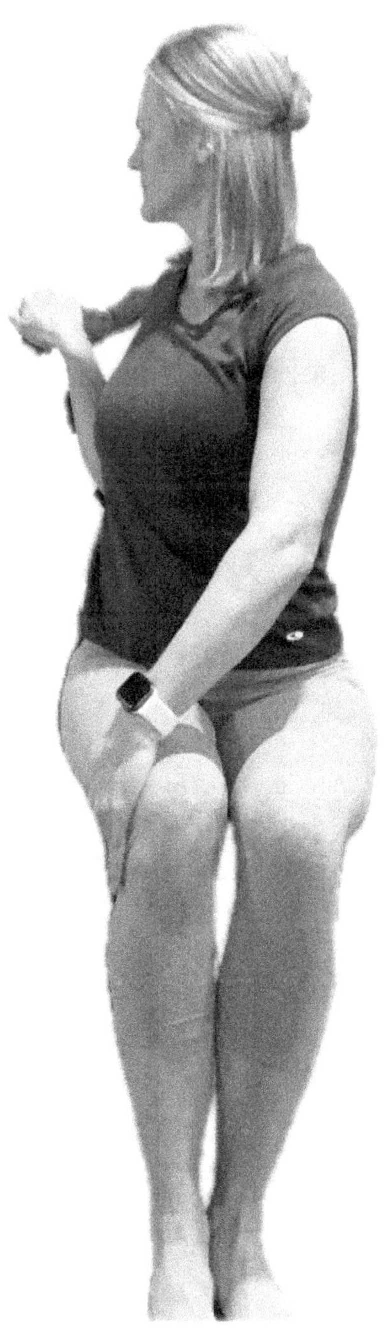

Seated Spinal Twist – Modifications:

- Instead of twisting the torso deeply, individuals with back issues can perform a gentler rotation, focusing on maintaining good spinal alignment.
- Use the chair's backrest for support if needed, avoiding any strain in the lower back or hips.

**Seated Side Bend:**

- Sit tall in your chair with your feet flat on the floor and your hands resting on your thighs.
- Inhale to lengthen your spine, then exhale as you lean to the right, sliding your right hand down your right thigh.
- Keep your left hand reaching towards the ceiling, feeling the stretch along the left side of your torso.
- Hold the stretch for a few breaths, engaging your core to support your spine.
- Inhale to return to center, then repeat on the other side.
- Aim for 3–5 repetitions on each side, moving with your breath.

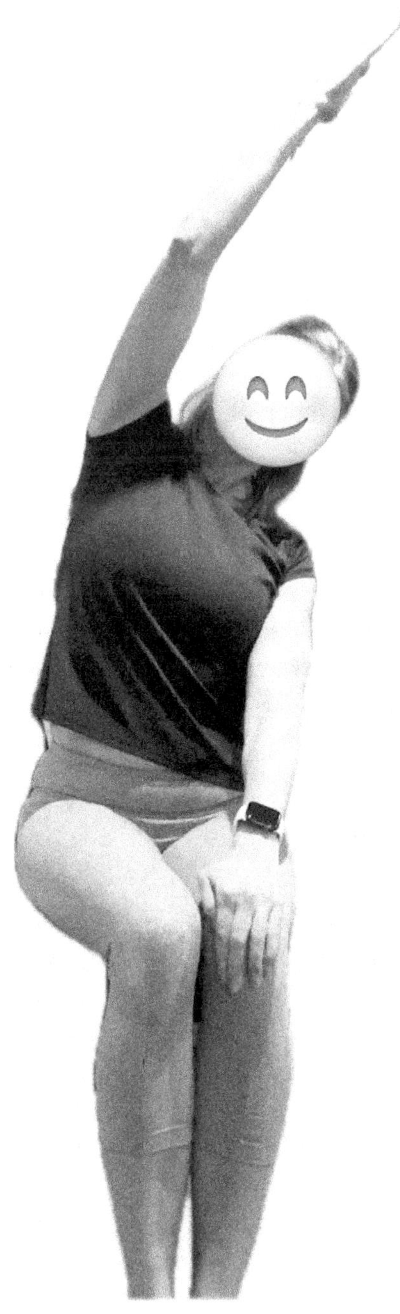

Seated Side Bend – Modifications:

- Individuals with limited mobility or balance concerns can perform a smaller side bend, focusing on lengthening one side of the torso while keeping the opposite hip grounded.
- Use a chair with and armrest for support, if needed, ensuring stability throughout the movement.

**Seated Knee-to-Chest Stretch:**

- Sit tall in your chair with your feet flat on the floor.
- Inhale and hug your right knee towards your chest, exhale while wrapping your arms around your shin.
- Keep your left foot planted firmly on the floor and your spine tall.
- Hold the stretch for a few breaths, feeling the engagement in your core as you draw your knee towards your chest.
- Release and switch sides, hugging your left knee towards your chest.
- Aim for 3-5 repetitions on each side, breathing deeply and maintaining good posture throughout.

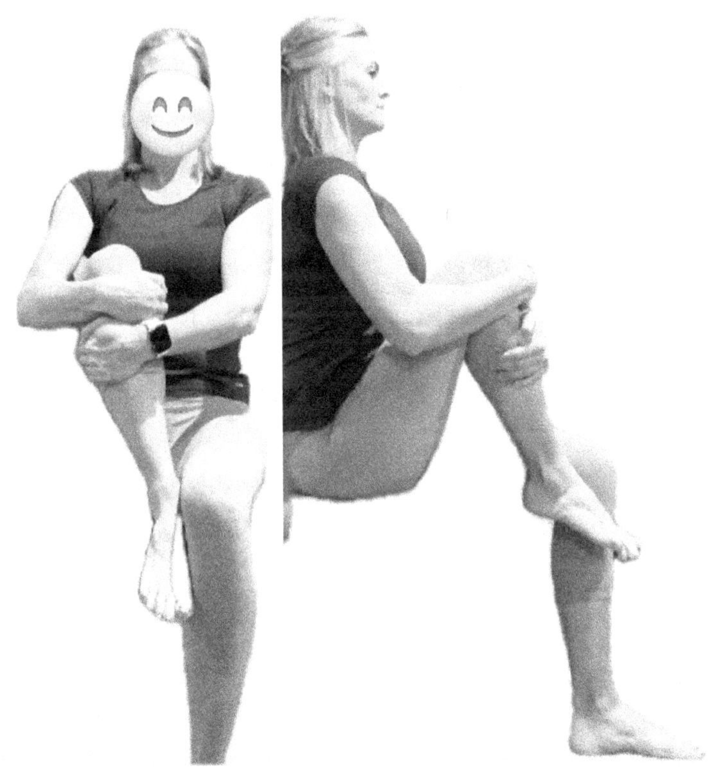

Seated Knee-to-Chest Stretch - Modifications:

- For individuals with knee or hip issues, limit the range of motion by hugging the knee towards the chest only as far as feels comfortable.
- Use the hands to support the leg if needed, avoiding any strain in the lower back or hips.
- Use a towel to wrap around the leg here as well to limit the strain on the low back or hips.

**Seated Boat Pose Variation:**

- Sit tall in your chair with your feet flat on the floor and your hands resting on your thighs.
- Inhale and engage your core muscles and lean back slightly, exhale while lifting your feet off the floor and balancing on your sit bones.
- Keep your knees bent and your shins parallel to the floor, finding a comfortable position that challenges your core without straining your lower back.
- Hold the pose for a few breaths, focusing on maintaining stability and engagement in your core.
- Lower your feet back to the floor and rest for a moment before repeating.
- Aim for 3–5 repetitions, gradually increasing as you build strength and endurance.

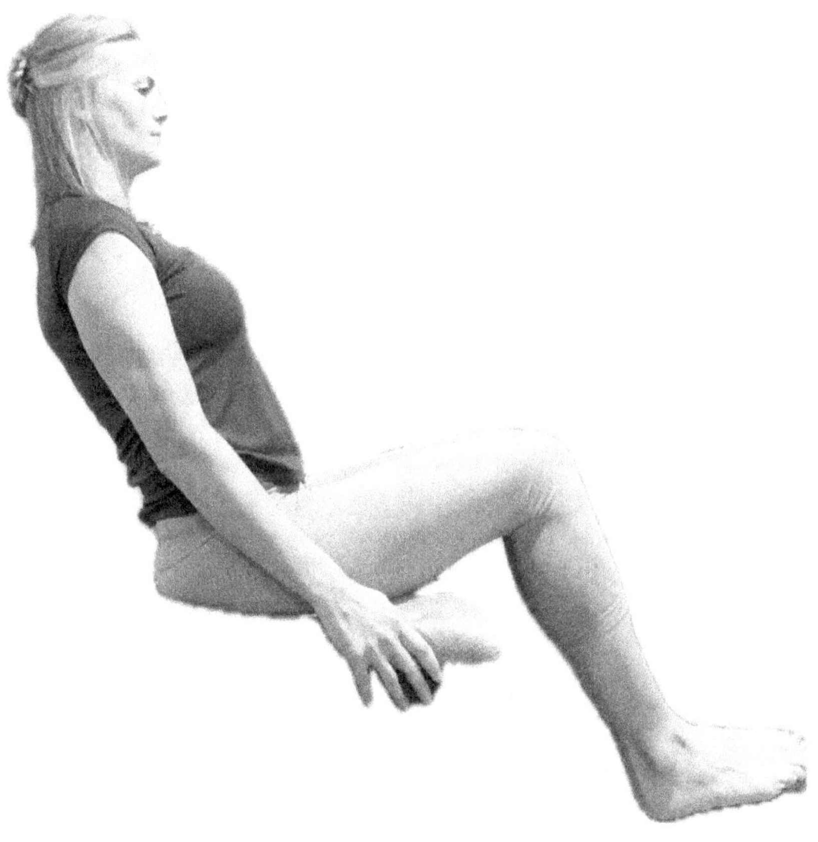

Seated Boat Pose – Modifications:

- If balancing on the sit bones is challenging, keep both feet flat on the floor and focus on engaging the core muscles while lifting one foot at a time.
- Use the chair's backrest for support if needed, ensuring stability throughout the movement.

Incorporate these gentle chair yoga poses and stretches into your routine to strengthen your core muscles effectively without straining your body. Focus on moving mindfully, breathing deeply, and maintaining proper alignment to maximize the benefits of each exercise while minimizing the risk of injury. With consistent practice, you can build core strength, improve stability, and support overall spinal health for greater comfort and mobility. By implementing these modifications, individuals with arthritis or other physical limitations can safely and comfortably practice chair yoga, enjoying the benefits of improved flexibility, strength, and overall well-being. It's essential to listen to the body, honor its limitations, and adjust the practice as needed to ensure a positive and enjoyable experience.

**Breathing Techniques for Relaxation and Vitality**

The breath is a powerful tool for relaxation and vitality, serving as a bridge between body and mind. By incorporating breathing techniques into your chair yoga practice, you can promote relaxation, reduce stress, and increase energy levels. From deep belly breathing to alternate nostril breathing, these techniques offer a simple yet effective way to enhance your overall well-being.

Effective breathing techniques can serve as powerful tools for promoting relaxation, reducing stress, and boosting vitality. Incorporating breathwork into your chair yoga practice can help calm the mind, energize the body, and enhance overall well-being. Here are some simple yet effective breathing techniques to try:

Deep Belly Breathing (Diaphragmatic Breathing):

- Sit comfortably in your chair with your feet flat on the floor and your hands resting on your thighs.
- Close your eyes and take a few slow, deep breaths, inhaling through

your nose and exhaling through your mouth to release tension.
- Place one hand on your abdomen and one hand on your chest.
- Inhale deeply through your nose, allowing your abdomen to expand fully as you fill your lungs with air. Feel your hand rise as your belly expands.
- Exhale slowly and completely through your mouth, allowing your abdomen to contract as you release the breath. Feel your hand lower as your belly deflates.
- Continue this deep belly breathing pattern for several breaths, focusing on the sensation of your breath moving in and out of your body.

Equal Breathing:

- Sit comfortably in your chair with your spine tall and your hands resting on your thighs.
- Close your eyes and take a few natural breaths to center yourself.
- Inhale slowly and deeply through your nose for a count of four counts.
- Exhale slowly and completely through your nose for a count of four counts, matching the duration of your inhalation.
- Continue this equal breathing pattern for several rounds, maintaining a steady rhythm and focusing on the evenness of your breath.

Alternate Nostril Breathing:

- Sit comfortably in your chair with your spine tall and your hands resting on your thighs.
- Use your right thumb to close your right nostril and inhale deeply

through your left nostril.

- Use your right ring finger to close your left nostril and exhale completely through your right nostril.
- Inhale deeply through your right nostril, then close it with your right thumb and exhale through your left nostril.
- Continue this alternate nostril breathing pattern for several rounds, focusing on the smooth transition between inhales and exhales and maintaining a relaxed pace.

Lion's Breath:

- Sit comfortably in your chair with your spine tall and your hands resting on your thighs.
- Inhale deeply through your nose, filling your lungs with air.
- Exhale forcefully through your mouth, sticking out your tongue and making a "ha" sound as you exhale, as if you were a lion roaring.
- Repeat this lion's breath for several rounds, allowing yourself to release tension and pent-up energy with each exhale.

Relaxing Breath (4-7-8 Breathing):

- Sit comfortably in your chair with your spine tall and your hands resting on your thighs.
- Inhale deeply through your nose for a count of four counts.
- Hold your breath at the top of the inhale for a count of seven counts.
- Exhale slowly and completely through your mouth for a count of eight counts, making a whooshing sound as you release the breath.
- Repeat this 4-7-8 breathing pattern for several rounds, allowing yourself to sink deeper into relaxation with each exhale.

Choose one or more of these breathing techniques to incorporate into your chair yoga practice, depending on your preferences and needs. Practice regularly to experience the calming and revitalizing effects of conscious breathing, supporting your overall well-being and vitality.

**Short and Sweet: 10 Minute Routine for Busy Days**

In today's fast-paced world, finding time for self-care can be a challenge. That's why we've included a series of short and sweet 10-minute routines designed for busy days. Whether you're at home or in the office, these quick practices offer a convenient way to sneak in some self-care and rejuvenation.

When time is limited, a brief yet effective chair yoga routine can provide a refreshing break and rejuvenate the body and mind. Here's a 10-minute routine that targets the whole body (I have included pictures where the poses have not been previously described):

**Seated Mountain Pose (1 minute):**

- Sit tall in your chair with your feet flat on the floor and your hands resting on your thighs.
- Close your eyes and take a few deep breaths, grounding yourself in the present moment.
- Engage your core muscles and lengthen your spine, imagining yourself as a steady mountain.

**Seated Cat-Cow Stretch (1 minute):**

- Inhale as you arch your back, lifting your chest and gaze towards the ceiling (Cow Pose).
- Exhale as you round your spine, tucking your chin towards your

chest and drawing your belly button towards your spine (Cat Pose).

- Flow between Cat and Cow Poses with your breath for several rounds, gently warming up the spine.

**Seated Forward Fold (1 minute):**

- Inhale as you lengthen your spine, reaching your arms overhead.
- Exhale as you hinge forward from your hips, folding forward and reaching towards your feet or the floor.
- Hold the stretch for a few breaths, feeling the lengthening sensation along your spine and the back of your legs.

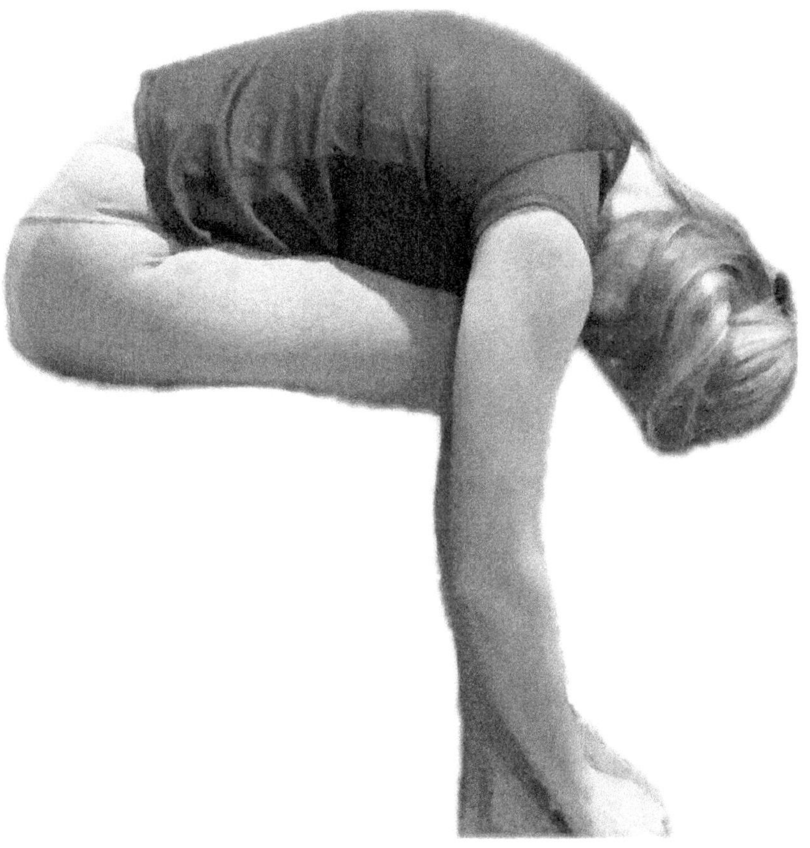

**Seated Spinal Twist (1 minute each side):**

- Inhale to lengthen your spine, then exhale as you twist your torso to the right, placing your left hand on the outside of your right thigh and your right hand on the back of the chair.
- Hold the twist for a few breaths, feeling the gentle rotation in your spine.

- Inhale to return to center, then repeat on the other side.

**Seated Knee-to-Chest Stretch (1 minute each side):**

- Hug your right knee towards your chest, wrapping your arms around your shin.
- Hold the stretch for a few breaths, feeling the release in your lower back and hips.
- Release and switch sides, hugging your left knee towards your chest.

**Seated Side Bend (1 minute each side):**

- Inhale to lengthen your spine, then exhale as you lean to the right, sliding your right hand down your right thigh and reaching your left arm overhead.
- Hold the stretch for a few breaths, feeling the lengthening sensation along the left side of your torso.
- Inhale to return to center, then repeat on the other side.

**Seated Relaxation Pose (2 minutes):**

- Sit comfortably in your chair with your feet flat on the floor and your hands resting on your thighs.
- Close your eyes and take several deep breaths, allowing your body to relax completely.
- Release any tension in your muscles and let go of any lingering thoughts or worries.

This 10-minute chair yoga routine provides a balanced combination of stretches, twists, and relaxation techniques to invigorate the body and calm the mind, making it perfect for busy days when time is limited.

Practice regularly to reap the benefits of improved flexibility, mobility, and overall well-being.

**Advanced: Balance Poses Using a Chair for Support**

For those seeking a greater challenge, balance poses offer an opportunity to refine stability and focus. With the support of a chair, you can explore advanced balance poses with confidence and ease. From tree pose to warrior III, these poses challenge both body and mind, fostering a deeper sense of strength and resilience.

As we explore the world of chair yoga poses, remember to listen to your body and honor its needs. With regular practice and mindful awareness, you can experience the transformative power of yoga from the comfort of your own chair.

Balance poses are excellent for improving stability, coordination, and proprioception, especially for seniors. Using a chair for support adds an extra layer of safety and confidence, allowing individuals to challenge themselves while maintaining stability. Here are some advanced balance poses using a chair for support:

**Chair Tree Pose:**

- Stand behind a chair with your feet hip-width apart and your hands resting lightly on the backrest for support.
- Shift your weight into your left foot and lift your right foot off the ground, placing the sole of your right foot against your left inner thigh or calf (avoid the knee).
- Engage your core muscles and lengthen your spine, finding a focal point to help maintain balance.
- Hold the pose for several breaths, feeling rooted through your standing foot and extending through your spine and crown.

- Repeat on the other side, balancing on your right foot and placing your left foot against your right inner thigh or calf.

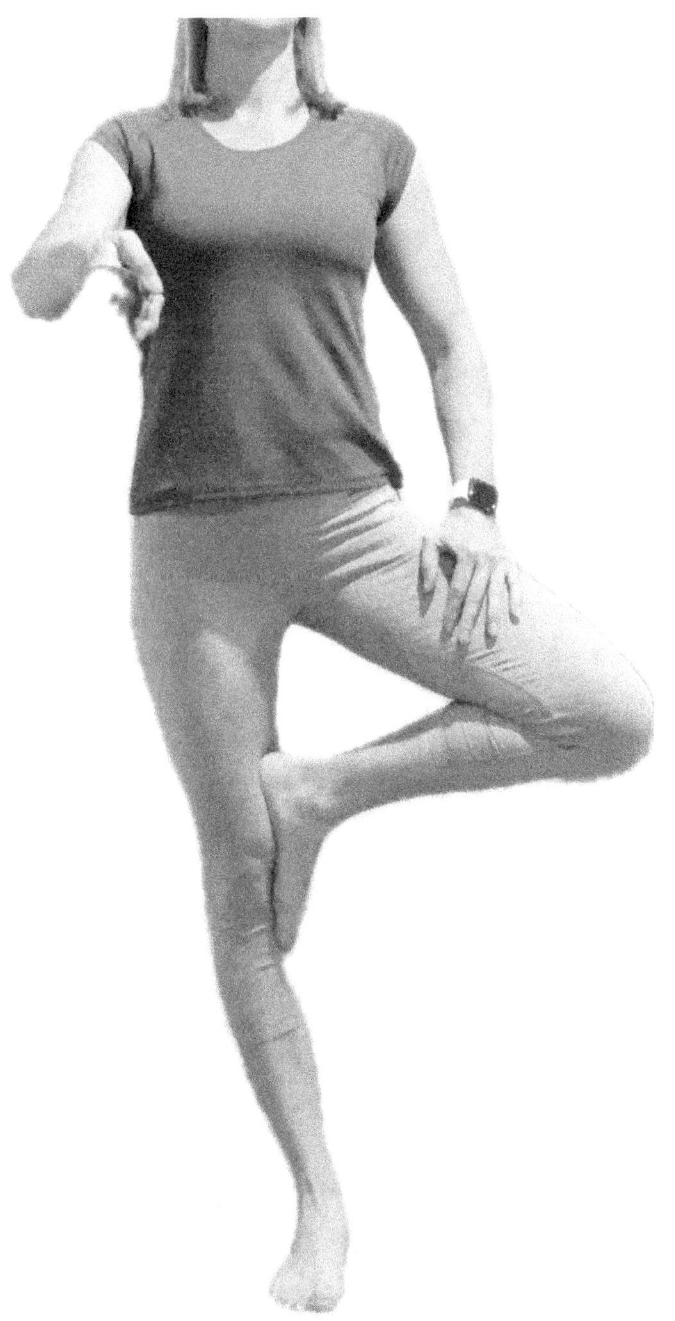

**Chair Warrior III Pose:**

- Stand behind a chair with your feet hip-width apart and your hands resting lightly on the backrest for support.
- Shift your weight into your left foot and hinge forward from your hips, extending your right leg straight behind you and parallel to the floor.
- Keep your hips squared towards the chair and your torso parallel to the floor, reaching your arms forward alongside your ears for balance.
- Engage your core muscles and lengthen through your extended leg and spine, creating a straight line from your head to your heel.
- Hold the pose for several breaths, focusing on stability and alignment.
- Repeat on the other side, balancing on your right foot and extending your left leg behind you.

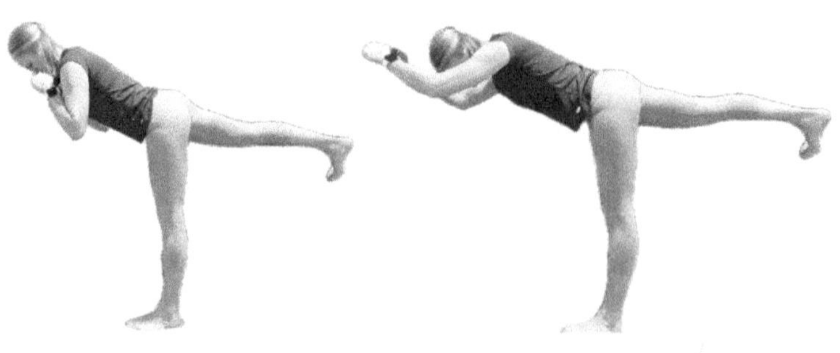

**Chair Extended Hand-to-Big-Toe Pose:**

- Stand beside a chair with your feet hip-width apart and your right hand resting lightly on the backrest for support.
- Shift your weight into your left foot and lift your right foot off the ground, bending your right knee and bringing it towards your chest.
- Reach down with your right hand and grasp the big toe of your right foot, extending your leg straight out in front of you.
- Engage your core muscles and lengthen through your spine, finding balance and stability.
- Hold the pose for several breaths, focusing on the extension through your raised leg and the engagement of your standing leg.
- Repeat on the other side, balancing on your right foot and extending your left leg in front of you.

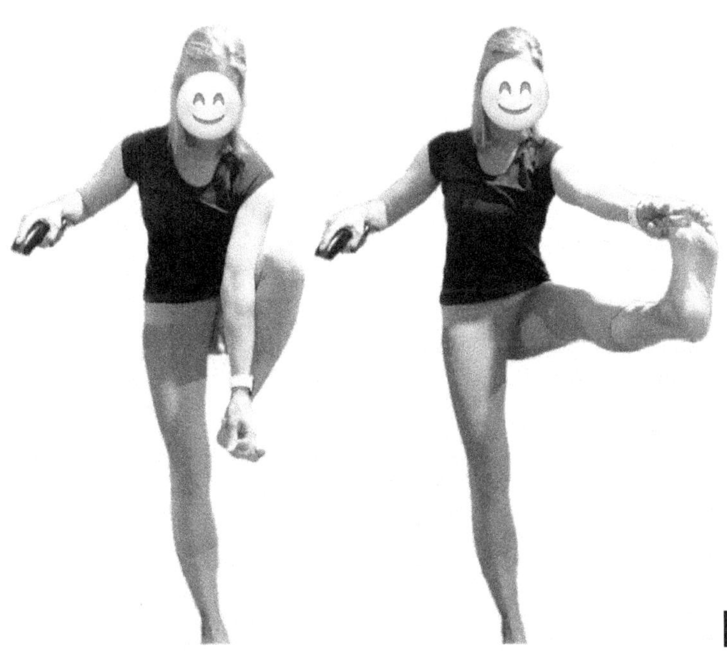

**Chair Eagle Pose:**

- Stand behind a chair with your feet hip-width apart and your hands resting lightly on the backrest for support.
- Shift your weight into your left foot and cross your right thigh over your left thigh, wrapping your right foot around your left calf if possible.
- Bend your knees slightly and cross your left elbow over your right elbow, bringing your palms together if accessible.
- Engage your core muscles and lengthen through your spine, finding stability and balance in the pose.
- Hold the pose for several breaths, focusing on the alignment of your crossed limbs and the engagement of your core.
- Repeat on the other side, crossing your left thigh over your right thigh and your right elbow over your left elbow.

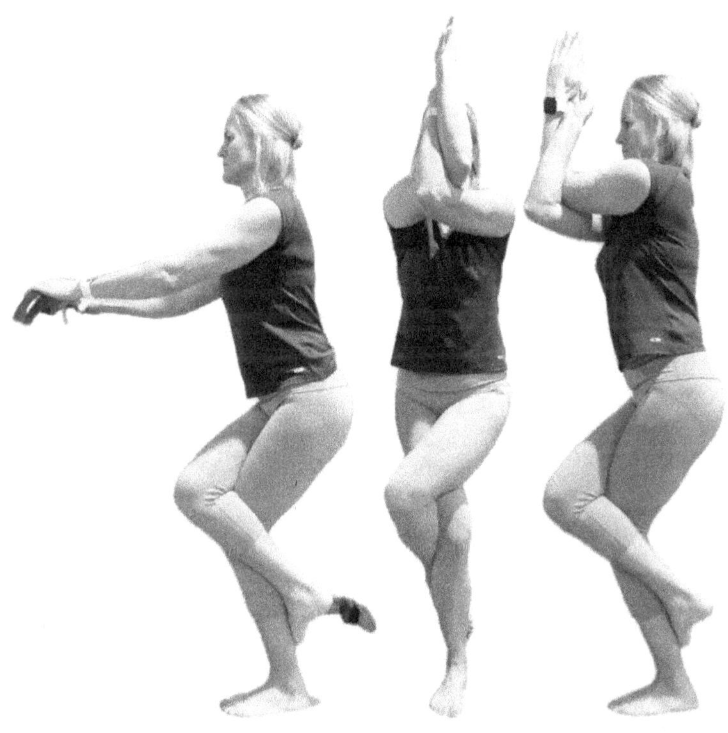

Practice these advanced balance poses using a chair for support to challenge your stability, improve your coordination, and enhance your overall sense of well-being. As you become more comfortable with the poses, you can gradually decrease your reliance on the chair for support and explore balancing without assistance. Remember to listen to your body, honor its limitations, and adjust the poses as needed to ensure safety and comfort.

5

# Addressing Common Senior Health Concerns

I n the pursuit of holistic wellness, chair yoga serves as a powerful tool for addressing common health concerns that seniors may face. From joint pain to mental health, this chapter explores how specific yoga poses can directly impact and alleviate these issues, promoting overall well-being and vitality.

**Chair Yoga for Joint Relief and Arthritis**

Joint pain and arthritis are prevalent concerns among seniors, often hindering mobility and quality of life. Through gentle and targeted chair yoga poses, individuals can find relief from stiffness and inflammation, improving range of motion and joint flexibility. From wrist circles to knee lifts, these poses offer a gentle yet effective way to nourish and support the joints.

Chair yoga offers gentle movements and stretches that can help alleviate joint discomfort and improve flexibility for individuals with arthritis. By incorporating specific poses into your practice, you can target affected joints and promote greater mobility and comfort. Here are examples of some previously discussed poses and how they benefit arthritic joints:

Seated Cat-Cow Stretch:

- This gentle spinal movement helps lubricate the joints of the spine, including those affected by arthritis.
- The rhythmic flexion and extension of the spine can improve flexibility and reduce stiffness in the back, neck, and shoulders.
- Seated Shoulder Stretch:
- Stretching the shoulders and upper back can alleviate tension and stiffness in the joints, common symptoms of arthritis.
- This pose promotes better range of motion in the shoulder joints and helps prevent the development of frozen shoulder.

Seated Knee-to-Chest Stretch:

- By bringing the knee towards the chest, this pose helps increase flexibility in the hip and knee joints.
- It can also provide relief for arthritic hips by gently stretching the muscles and connective tissue surrounding the joint.

Seated Spinal Twist:

- Twisting poses like this one help improve mobility in the spine and promote healthy rotation of the vertebrae.
- The twisting action can also stimulate circulation and reduce inflammation in the joints, including those affected by arthritis.

Seated Forward Fold:

- This pose stretches the hamstrings and lower back, relieving tension and discomfort in the lumbar spine and hips.

- It can also help alleviate stiffness in the knees and improve circulation to the lower extremities.

Chair Tree Pose:

- Balancing poses like Tree Pose help strengthen the muscles surrounding the joints and improve stability and proprioception.
- By challenging balance and coordination, this pose can also help prevent falls, which can be particularly concerning for individuals with arthritis.

Chair Warrior III Pose:

- Warrior III strengthens the muscles of the legs, hips, and core, providing stability and support for arthritic joints.
- The pose also encourages proper alignment and posture, reducing strain on the joints and promoting overall joint health.

Chair Extended Hand-to-Big-Toe Pose:

- Stretching the hamstrings and calves in this pose can relieve tension and discomfort in the knees and ankles.
- By improving flexibility in the lower body, this pose can help reduce stiffness and pain associated with arthritis.

Incorporate these chair yoga poses into your daily practice to experience relief from joint discomfort and improve flexibility and mobility in arthritic joints. Listen to your body, and modify the poses as needed to ensure comfort and safety. With consistent practice, you can cultivate greater ease and well-being in your body, even with arthritis.

## Boosting Cardiovascular Health with Gentle Movement

Maintaining cardiovascular health is essential for overall vitality and longevity. Chair yoga poses that incorporate gentle movement and breathwork can help improve circulation, lower blood pressure, and strengthen the heart. From seated sun salutations to gentle twists, these poses offer a heart-healthy way to promote cardiovascular wellness.

Chair yoga offers a low-impact way to promote cardiovascular health through gentle movements that improve circulation, reduce blood pressure, and support heart health. Several studies have explored the effects of chair yoga on cardiovascular parameters, demonstrating its positive impact on overall cardiovascular well-being. Here are some studies that highlight the benefits of chair yoga for heart health:

Study 1:

- Research: A study published in the Journal of Geriatric Physical Therapy investigated the effects of a 12-week chair yoga program on cardiovascular health in older adults.
- Findings: The study found significant improvements in participants' blood pressure, heart rate variability, and arterial stiffness after completing the chair yoga program. These improvements indicate better cardiovascular function and reduced risk of cardiovascular disease.

Study 2:

- Research: Another study published in the Journal of Alternative and Complementary Medicine examined the effects of chair yoga on cardiovascular risk factors in sedentary older adults with hypertension.
- Findings: The study reported reductions in systolic and diastolic

blood pressure among participants who practiced chair yoga regularly. Additionally, improvements in heart rate variability and lipid profiles were observed, indicating a lower risk of cardiovascular events.

Study 3:

- Research: A randomized controlled trial published in the American Journal of Health Promotion compared the effects of chair yoga and aerobic exercise on cardiovascular health in older adults.
- Findings: The study found that both chair yoga and aerobic exercise led to improvements in cardiovascular fitness, with chair yoga showing comparable benefits to aerobic exercise. Participants in the chair yoga group experienced reductions in blood pressure and improvements in heart rate variability, indicating enhanced cardiovascular function.

These studies demonstrate the significant impact of chair yoga on cardiovascular health, including improvements in circulation, blood pressure, and heart rate variability. By incorporating gentle movement and breathwork into daily practice, individuals can support their heart health and reduce their risk of cardiovascular disease. Regular participation in chair yoga can contribute to overall well-being and enhance quality of life for individuals of all ages, especially seniors seeking to maintain cardiovascular health.

**Yoga for Mental Health: Combatting Anxiety and Depression**

Mental health concerns such as anxiety and depression can significantly impact quality of life and overall well-being. Chair yoga provides a safe and supportive environment for individuals to explore mindfulness and relaxation techniques, promoting mental clarity and emotional balance. Through calming breathwork and grounding poses, individuals can cultivate a sense of peace and resilience in the face of adversity.

Chair yoga not only benefits physical health but also plays a crucial role in promoting mental well-being by alleviating symptoms of anxiety and depression. Engaging in chair yoga triggers various physiological and psychological mechanisms within the body that contribute to improved mental health. Here's how chair yoga helps combat anxiety and depression and promotes overall mental well-being:

Stress Reduction and Relaxation:

- Chair yoga incorporates deep breathing exercises and relaxation techniques, such as mindfulness and meditation, which activate the parasympathetic nervous system. This induces a relaxation response in the body, reducing stress hormones like cortisol and promoting a sense of calm and tranquility.

Release of Endorphins:

- Practicing chair yoga stimulates the release of endorphins, which are neurotransmitters that act as natural painkillers and mood elevators. Endorphins help reduce feelings of anxiety and depression, promoting a sense of well-being and happiness.

Mind-Body Connection:

- Chair yoga emphasizes the mind-body connection, encouraging individuals to focus on their breath, body sensations, and present moment awareness. This mindfulness practice increases self-awareness and emotional regulation, helping individuals manage symptoms of anxiety and depression more effectively.

Improvement in Sleep Quality:

- Chair yoga promotes relaxation and stress reduction, which can lead to improved sleep quality. Better sleep patterns contribute to overall mental health by reducing symptoms of anxiety and depression and enhancing cognitive function and emotional resilience.

Social Interaction and Support:

- Participating in chair yoga classes provides opportunities for social interaction and support, which are essential for mental well-being. Connecting with others in a supportive environment can reduce feelings of loneliness and isolation, common risk factors for anxiety and depression.

Enhanced Self-Efficacy and Empowerment:

- Chair yoga encourages individuals to listen to their bodies, honor their limitations, and celebrate their progress. This fosters a sense of self-efficacy and empowerment, empowering individuals to take control of their mental health and well-being.

By engaging in chair yoga regularly, individuals can cultivate a greater sense of peace, resilience, and emotional balance, making it an effective tool for combating anxiety and depression. Through mindful movement, breathwork, and relaxation techniques, chair yoga promotes holistic well-being and supports mental health in individuals of all ages and abilities.

**Improving Sleep Quality through Relaxation Techniques**

Quality sleep is essential for physical and mental rejuvenation, yet many seniors struggle with insomnia and sleep disturbances. Chair yoga poses that focus on relaxation and stress reduction can help promote restful sleep and improve overall sleep quality. From gentle stretches to guided relaxation exercises, these poses offer a tranquil way to unwind and prepare for a restorative night's sleep.

**Chair Yoga for Digestive Health**

Digestive issues such as bloating, constipation, and indigestion are common concerns among seniors, often stemming from sedentary lifestyles and poor dietary habits. Chair yoga poses that incorporate gentle twists and forward folds can help stimulate digestion, improve circulation to the digestive organs, and alleviate discomfort. From seated twists to belly breathing exercises, these poses offer a natural and gentle way to support digestive health.

**Enhancing Respiratory Health with Pranayama**

Respiratory health is vital for overall well-being, yet many seniors experience diminished lung capacity and respiratory function with age. Chair yoga poses that focus on deep breathing and pranayama techniques can help strengthen the respiratory muscles, increase lung capacity, and improve oxygenation of the body. From diaphragmatic breathing to alternate nostril breathing, these practices offer a rejuvenating way to enhance respiratory health.

By incorporating specific chair yoga poses targeted towards common senior health concerns, individuals can experience relief, vitality, and resilience in body, mind, and spirit. Through regular practice and mindful awareness, chair yoga serves as a powerful tool for promoting overall well-being and enhancing quality of life.

6

# Nutrition and Lifestyle for Optimal Benefits

I n the pursuit of optimal health and well-being, nutrition plays a crucial role in supporting and enhancing our yoga practice, especially for seniors. This chapter explores the fundamental principles of nutrition and lifestyle choices that can complement and amplify the benefits of chair yoga.

**Hydration: The Key to Effective Exercise**

Hydration is essential for supporting physical activity and maintaining overall health, particularly as we age. Adequate hydration helps regulate body temperature, lubricate joints, and transport nutrients to cells, ensuring optimal function and performance during exercise. Lack of hydration has been linked to stiffness, fatigue, injury, lethargy and memory loss. Remember that the recommended daily intake is 64 ounces (or 8 small cups of water) per day.

**Superfoods for Seniors: Boosting Your Yoga Practice**

Nutrient-dense superfoods offer a powerhouse of vitamins, minerals, and antioxidants that can support and enhance our yoga practice. From leafy greens to omega-3-rich fish, incorporating superfoods into our diet can help promote energy, vitality, and overall well-being. This section will highlight a variety of superfoods that are particularly beneficial for seniors, along with creative ways to incorporate them into meals and snacks. Just by making small adjustments to your diet will impact your overall energy level and weight.

Seniors engaging in chair yoga can enhance their practice and overall well-being by incorporating nutrient-dense superfoods into their diets. These foods are packed with essential vitamins, minerals, antioxidants, and other nutrients that support optimal health, energy levels, and recovery. Here are examples of superfoods that seniors can benefit from, helping to boost their yoga practice:

Berries (e.g., blueberries, strawberries, raspberries):

- Berries are rich in antioxidants, particularly flavonoids, which help reduce inflammation and oxidative stress in the body.
- They support brain health, improve cognitive function, and may help protect against age-related cognitive decline.

Leafy Greens (e.g., spinach, kale, Swiss chard):

- Leafy greens are packed with vitamins A, C, and K, as well as folate, potassium, and fiber.
- They support heart health, bone health, and digestive health, while also providing essential nutrients for overall well-being.

Fatty Fish (e.g., salmon, mackerel, sardines):

- Fatty fish are excellent sources of omega-3 fatty acids, which have anti-inflammatory properties and support heart and brain health.

- They can help reduce the risk of cardiovascular disease, improve mood, and support cognitive function.

Nuts and Seeds (e.g., almonds, walnuts, chia seeds):

- Nuts and seeds are rich in healthy fats, protein, fiber, vitamins, and minerals.
- They provide sustained energy, support heart health, and help regulate blood sugar levels.

Yogurt and Fermented Foods (e.g., Greek yogurt, kefir, sauerkraut):

- Yogurt and fermented foods are rich in probiotics, beneficial bacteria that support gut health and digestion.
- They help maintain a healthy balance of gut flora, support immune function, and may improve mood and mental well-being.

Whole Grains (e.g., quinoa, brown rice, oats):

- Whole grains are high in fiber, vitamins, minerals, and antioxidants, providing sustained energy and promoting digestive health.
- They support heart health, help regulate blood sugar levels, and may reduce the risk of chronic diseases such as diabetes and cancer.

Turmeric:

- Turmeric contains curcumin, a powerful anti-inflammatory and antioxidant compound with numerous health benefits.
- It helps reduce inflammation, support joint health, and may improve cognitive function and mood.

Dark Chocolate:

- Dark chocolate is rich in antioxidants, particularly flavonoids, which have been shown to improve heart health and cognitive function.
- It may also help reduce stress, improve mood, and promote relaxation.

Incorporating these superfoods into a senior's diet can provide essential nutrients and support overall health and well-being, enhancing the benefits of their chair yoga practice. By nourishing the body with nutrient-dense foods, seniors can optimize their energy levels, support recovery, and promote longevity, allowing them to enjoy the physical and mental benefits of yoga to the fullest.

**The Importance of Rest and Recovery**

Rest and recovery are integral components of any exercise regimen, including chair yoga. Proper rest allows the body to repair and regenerate tissues, reduce inflammation, and replenish energy stores, ensuring optimal performance and preventing burnout or injury.

By prioritizing hydration, incorporating nutrient-dense superfoods into our diet, and embracing rest and recovery, seniors can optimize the benefits of chair yoga and enhance their overall health and well-being. As we continue our journey towards holistic wellness, let us nourish our bodies, minds, and spirits with mindful nutrition and lifestyle choices that support and sustain us on the path to optimal health.

7

# Conclusion

I truly hope that, as a beginner, you feel empowered that you have the tools to put together a safe yoga routine that fits your lifestyle. Congratulations on completing your journey through "Chair Yoga for Seniors: Reduce Stress, Lose Weight, and Increase Flexibility." By picking up this book, you've taken a significant step towards reclaiming your vitality and well-being, regardless of age or physical condition.

Throughout these pages, you've discovered the transformative power of chair yoga and learned how it can positively impact your life. From gentle stretches to mindful breathing exercises, you've gained valuable tools to enhance flexibility, mobility, and reduce stress in your daily life.

**Embracing the Journey:**

It's important to recognize that the path to bettering yourself is not always linear. Like any fitness journey, you may encounter ups and downs along the way. Remember that setbacks are natural and part of the process. Stay committed to yourself, trust in your abilities, and have patience with yourself as you navigate this journey.

Thank you for allowing me to be your guide on this journey. As you continue to integrate chair yoga into your life, may you find joy, peace, and vitality in every breath and movement. Remember, the power to transform your life lies within you. Keep practicing, stay committed, and embrace the journey ahead.

With gratitude.

Leave a Review: If you found this information helpful and transformative, I encourage you to leave a review on Amazon. Your feedback can help other potential readers discover the benefits of chair yoga and embark on their own journey towards wellness.